The Sweet Spot

Achieving Optimal Health Through Blood Sugar Balance

By

Louisiana Hades

Table of contents

Introduction

The Importance of Blood Sugar Balance for Optimal Health

The food we eat is the fuel that powers our bodies, and it all starts with glucose, a simple sugar that is our body's primary source of energy. However, while glucose is essential for life, too much of it can be harmful, leading to a range of health problems such as obesity, type 2 diabetes, and cardiovascular disease. This is why maintaining blood sugar balance is critical for optimal health.

Blood sugar balance refers to the level of glucose in our blood at any given time. When we eat carbohydrates, such as bread, pasta, or fruit, our body breaks them down into glucose, which enters our bloodstream. In response, our pancreas releases insulin, a hormone that helps move glucose from our bloodstream into our cells, where it can be used for energy or stored for later use.

However, when we eat too many carbohydrates or consume foods with a high glycemic index (a measure of how quickly a food raises blood glucose levels), our body can produce too much insulin. This can cause a rapid drop in blood sugar, leading to cravings, fatigue, and other symptoms, as well as long-term health problems if it happens repeatedly.

On the other hand, when we eat too few carbohydrates or consume foods with a low glycemic index, our body may not produce enough insulin, causing blood sugar to remain high for an extended period. This can also lead to health problems over time, as high blood sugar can damage blood vessels, nerves, and organs.

Therefore, maintaining blood sugar balance is crucial for optimal health. When our blood sugar is balanced, we feel more energized, our cravings are reduced, and our mood is more stable. Furthermore, maintaining balanced blood sugar levels can reduce our risk of developing chronic diseases such as type 2 diabetes, heart disease, and certain types of cancer.

Achieving and maintaining blood sugar balance requires a combination of healthy eating habits, regular exercise, and stress management techniques. In this book, we will explore the science of blood sugar balance, including how different foods affect blood sugar levels, how insulin works, and the impact of exercise and stress on blood sugar. We will also provide practical tips and strategies for achieving and maintaining blood sugar balance in daily life.

Overall, blood sugar balance is critical for optimal health, and understanding how to achieve and maintain it can have a profound impact on our well-being. By making simple changes to our diet and lifestyle, we can improve our energy, reduce our risk of chronic disease, and achieve a greater sense of balance and vitality in our lives.

Chapter 1

Understanding the Glycemic Index: How Different Foods Affect Blood Sugar Levels

The glycemic index (GI) is a measure of how quickly a carbohydrate-containing food raises blood glucose levels. The GI scale ranges from 0 to 100, with higher values indicating a more rapid increase in blood glucose levels. Understanding the GI of different foods can help us make informed choices about what we eat and maintain blood sugar balance.

Foods with a high GI are rapidly digested and absorbed, causing a rapid increase in blood glucose levels. Examples of high GI foods include white bread, white rice, sugary drinks, and candy. These foods can cause a quick spike in blood sugar, followed by a rapid drop, which can leave us feeling tired, irritable, and hungry soon after eating.

In contrast, foods with a low GI are more slowly digested and absorbed, leading to a slower and more gradual increase in blood glucose levels. Examples of low GI foods include whole grains, legumes, fruits, and vegetables. These foods provide a more sustained release of energy and can help us feel fuller for longer.

The GI of a food can also be affected by factors such as cooking time and processing. For example, overcooking pasta can increase its GI, while cooking rice with coconut oil and then cooling it can lower its GI.

It's important to note that the GI is not the only factor that affects blood sugar levels. The amount and type of carbohydrates, as well as the presence of protein, fat, and fiber in a meal, can all impact blood sugar levels. However, the GI can be a useful tool for understanding how different foods affect blood sugar and making more informed choices.

It's also worth noting that the GI is not a one-size-fits-all approach. Individual responses to different foods can vary, depending on factors such as genetics, age, and activity level. Additionally, combining foods with different GIs can also affect blood sugar levels. For example, combining high GI foods with protein, fat, or fiber can help slow the absorption of glucose into the bloodstream.

In summary, understanding the GI of different foods can help us make more informed choices about what we eat and maintain blood sugar balance. While the GI is not the only factor that affects blood sugar levels, it can be a useful tool for guiding our food choices. By choosing more low GI foods, combining them with protein, fat, and fiber, and avoiding high GI foods, we can help promote optimal health and vitality.

Chapter 2

The Science of Insulin: How Insulin Affects Blood Sugar and Health

Insulin is a hormone produced by the pancreas that plays a critical role in regulating blood sugar levels and maintaining overall health. When we eat carbohydrates, they are broken down into glucose, which enters the bloodstream. Insulin helps to transport glucose from the bloodstream into cells throughout the body, where it can be used for energy or stored for later use.

In people with type 1 diabetes, the pancreas does not produce insulin, so insulin must be administered through injections or an insulin pump. In people with type 2 diabetes, the pancreas produces insulin, but the body's cells become resistant to its effects, leading to high blood sugar levels.

Insulin resistance can also occur in people without diabetes, particularly those who are overweight or obese. Over time, insulin resistance can lead to type 2 diabetes, as well as other health complications such as heart disease, stroke, and kidney disease.

In addition to regulating blood sugar levels, insulin also plays a role in other aspects of health. For example, insulin helps to regulate fat metabolism and storage. When insulin levels are high, the body is more likely to store fat, while low insulin levels can promote the breakdown of fat for energy.

Insulin also affects appetite and satiety. When insulin levels are high, we tend to feel less hungry and more satisfied after eating, while low insulin levels can lead to increased hunger and overeating.

Factors such as diet, exercise, and stress can all affect insulin levels and sensitivity. Eating a diet high in processed foods and sugar can lead to insulin resistance and increased insulin levels, while eating a diet rich in whole foods and fiber can improve insulin sensitivity and lower insulin levels.

Exercise can also improve insulin sensitivity, as physical activity helps to increase glucose uptake by muscle cells. Stress can have a negative impact on insulin sensitivity, as cortisol, a stress hormone, can increase insulin resistance and promote the breakdown of muscle tissue.

In summary, insulin plays a critical role in regulating blood sugar levels and maintaining overall health. Insulin resistance, which can occur in people with and without diabetes, can have negative impacts on health, including an increased risk of type 2 diabetes, heart disease, and other complications. Diet, exercise, and stress management can all play a role in improving insulin sensitivity and promoting optimal health.

Chapter 3

The Link Between Blood Sugar Balance and Weight Management

Blood sugar balance plays a crucial role in weight management, as it affects both hunger and metabolism. When blood sugar levels are too high, the body releases insulin to transport glucose from the bloodstream into cells. Insulin also promotes fat storage, which can lead to weight gain if blood sugar levels remain consistently elevated.

Conversely, when blood sugar levels drop too low, the body can enter a state of hypoglycemia, which can lead to increased hunger and overeating. This can create a cycle of blood sugar spikes and crashes, which can contribute to weight gain and difficulty losing weight.

Maintaining stable blood sugar levels throughout the day is key to promoting weight management. This can be achieved through a balanced diet that includes protein, healthy fats, and complex carbohydrates that are digested more slowly than simple carbohydrates. Eating smaller, frequent meals can also help to stabilize blood sugar levels and prevent overeating.

Exercise is another important component of blood sugar balance and weight management. Physical activity helps to increase glucose uptake by muscle cells, which can lead to lower blood sugar levels and improved insulin sensitivity. Exercise also helps to burn calories and promote weight loss.

Stress management is also important for blood sugar balance and weight management. Stress can increase cortisol levels, which can lead to increased insulin resistance and fat storage. Techniques such as meditation, deep breathing, and yoga can help to reduce stress and improve blood sugar balance.

In addition to promoting weight loss, blood sugar balance can also help to prevent weight gain and promote weight maintenance. By stabilizing blood sugar levels, individuals may experience fewer cravings and feel more satiated after meals, which can lead to consuming fewer calories overall.

However, it is important to note that weight management is a complex issue that can be influenced by a variety of factors beyond blood sugar balance, including genetics, sleep, and medication use. Consulting with a healthcare professional or registered dietitian can help to develop a personalized plan for achieving and maintaining a healthy weight.

In summary, blood sugar balance plays a critical role in weight management, affecting both hunger and metabolism. Eating a balanced diet, engaging in regular physical activity, and managing stress can all help to promote stable blood sugar levels and support weight management. However, weight management is a complex issue that may require individualized approaches for long-term success.

Chapter 4

The Role of Exercise in Maintaining Healthy Blood Sugar Levels

Exercise is a powerful tool for maintaining healthy blood sugar levels. When you exercise, your muscles use glucose for energy, which can help to lower your blood sugar levels. Exercise also increases insulin sensitivity, allowing your body to use insulin more efficiently and lower your blood sugar levels even further.

The benefits of exercise on blood sugar control are not limited to those with diabetes. Individuals with prediabetes or those at risk for developing diabetes can also benefit from regular exercise in preventing or delaying the onset of diabetes.

The type, duration, and intensity of exercise can all influence blood sugar levels. Aerobic exercise, such as brisk walking, cycling, or swimming, can help to lower blood sugar levels by increasing glucose uptake by the muscles. Resistance training, such as weight lifting, can also be effective in improving blood sugar control by increasing muscle mass and improving insulin sensitivity.

The American Diabetes Association recommends at least 150 minutes of moderate to vigorous intensity exercise per week, spread out over at least three days per week. This can be achieved through a variety of activities, such as walking, cycling, swimming, or strength training.

However, it is important to note that exercise can also cause blood sugar levels to drop too low, especially in individuals with diabetes who take insulin or other blood sugar-lowering medications. This is known as hypoglycemia and can cause symptoms such as dizziness, confusion, and even loss of consciousness. It is important to monitor blood sugar levels before, during, and after exercise and to consult with a healthcare professional before starting an exercise program.

In addition to improving blood sugar control, exercise has numerous other health benefits, such as improving cardiovascular health, reducing stress, and promoting weight loss. Regular exercise can also improve mood and energy levels, leading to an overall improved quality of life.

In summary, exercise is a powerful tool for maintaining healthy blood sugar levels. Aerobic exercise and resistance training can both be effective in improving blood sugar control, and the American Diabetes Association recommends at least 150 minutes of moderate to vigorous intensity exercise per week. However, it is important to monitor blood sugar levels and consult with a healthcare professional before starting an exercise program, especially for those with diabetes or at risk for developing diabetes. Regular exercise has numerous other health benefits, making it a crucial component of a healthy lifestyle.

Chapter 5

The Impact of Stress on Blood Sugar and Health

Stress is an unavoidable part of life, but when left unchecked, it can have a significant impact on our health, including our blood sugar levels. When we are under stress, our body releases hormones such as cortisol and adrenaline, which can cause a rise in blood sugar levels. This is known as the "fight or flight" response, which is a natural physiological response to stress.

While the occasional stressor may not have a significant impact on blood sugar levels, chronic or long-term stress can lead to consistently elevated blood sugar levels. This can have negative consequences for our health, as high blood sugar levels over time can damage organs and tissues throughout the body.

Chronic stress can also lead to a variety of other health problems, including high blood pressure, heart disease, and depression. Stress can also contribute to weight gain, as many people turn to food as a coping mechanism when under stress. This can further exacerbate blood sugar control issues and increase the risk of developing type 2 diabetes.

Furthermore, stress can also impact our sleep patterns, leading to sleep deprivation or poor quality sleep. This can also have negative effects on blood sugar control, as sleep deprivation has been shown to lead to insulin resistance and impaired glucose tolerance.

Fortunately, there are strategies that can help to mitigate the impact of stress on blood sugar and overall health. One of the most effective ways to reduce stress is through regular exercise. Exercise has been shown to reduce stress hormones and improve mood, which can have a positive impact on blood sugar levels.

Other stress-reducing strategies include mindfulness practices such as meditation or yoga, spending time in nature, and engaging in hobbies or activities that bring joy and relaxation. It is also important to maintain a healthy diet and get enough sleep, as these factors can also impact blood sugar control and overall health.

For those who are experiencing chronic stress or anxiety, it may be helpful to seek support from a mental health professional or counselor. They can provide tools and strategies to help manage stress and improve overall well-being.

In summary, stress can have a significant impact on blood sugar levels and overall health. Chronic stress can lead to consistently elevated blood sugar levels and contribute to a variety of health problems. However, there are strategies that can help to mitigate the impact of stress, including regular exercise, mindfulness practices, and seeking support from a mental health professional. By prioritizing stress management and self-care, we can improve our blood sugar control and overall health.

Chapter 6

Mindful Eating: A Tool for Achieving Blood Sugar Balance

Eating is a fundamental part of our lives, providing us with the fuel and nutrients we need to survive and thrive. However, many of us have lost touch with the experience of eating, often consuming our meals on the go or while distracted by technology or other tasks. This can lead to overeating, poor food choices, and ultimately, imbalanced blood sugar levels.

Mindful eating is an approach to eating that emphasizes being fully present and aware during the eating experience. It involves paying attention to the taste, smell, texture, and sensations of food, as well as our own hunger and satiety signals. By practicing mindful eating, we can better understand our body's needs and make choices that support balanced blood sugar levels.

One of the key principles of mindful eating is to eat slowly and without distractions. This allows us to fully savor the experience of eating and tune in to our body's signals of hunger and fullness. When we eat quickly or while distracted, we are more likely to overeat and consume foods that are high in sugar and refined carbohydrates, which can lead to blood sugar spikes and crashes.

Another important aspect of mindful eating is paying attention to the nutritional content of our food choices. This includes choosing whole, nutrient-dense foods that provide a balance of protein, healthy fats, and complex carbohydrates. These types of foods are digested more slowly, which can help to maintain stable blood sugar levels over time.

Mindful eating can also help us to recognize emotional triggers for eating, such as stress or boredom. By tuning in to our emotional state before we eat, we can make more conscious choices about what and how much we eat. This can help to prevent overeating and emotional eating, which can disrupt blood sugar balance.

Practicing mindful eating may seem daunting at first, but there are simple steps we can take to incorporate this approach into our daily lives. One strategy is to start small, such as taking a few deep breaths before beginning a meal or snack. This can help to center our attention and focus on the present moment.

Another strategy is to practice gratitude before eating, acknowledging the effort and energy that went into preparing the food and expressing appreciation for the nourishment it provides. This can help to shift our mindset from mindless consumption to mindful appreciation.

In addition to these techniques, it can be helpful to set aside dedicated time for meals and snacks, and to eat in a calm and peaceful environment. This can help to reduce distractions and allow us to fully engage with the eating experience.

In conclusion, mindful eating is a powerful tool for achieving blood sugar balance and overall health. By being fully present and aware during the eating experience, we can make more conscious choices about what and how much we eat, and better tune in to our body's needs. Incorporating mindful eating practices into our daily lives may take some effort, but the benefits can be profound, including improved blood sugar control, better digestion, and a greater sense of well-being.

Chapter 7

The Role of Fiber in Blood Sugar Regulation and Overall Health

Fiber is a type of carbohydrate that our bodies cannot digest or absorb. Despite this, it plays a crucial role in our health, including blood sugar regulation. Fiber comes in two forms: soluble and insoluble. Soluble fiber dissolves in water and forms a gel-like substance in the gut, while insoluble fiber does not dissolve and adds bulk to stool. Both types of fiber have important health benefits.

One of the key ways in which fiber helps regulate blood sugar levels is by slowing down the absorption of glucose into the bloodstream. When we eat foods that are high in refined carbohydrates, such as white bread or sugary drinks, the glucose is rapidly absorbed into the bloodstream, leading to a spike in blood sugar levels. This can cause a release of insulin, which can cause blood sugar levels to drop quickly, leading to fatigue, hunger, and cravings for more sugary foods. However, when we consume foods that are high in fiber, such as vegetables, fruits, and whole grains, the absorption of glucose is slowed down. This leads to a more gradual and sustained release of glucose into the bloodstream, which can help to maintain stable blood sugar levels over time.

In addition to its impact on blood sugar levels, fiber has a number of other health benefits. Soluble fiber, in particular, has been shown to lower cholesterol levels by binding to bile acids in the gut and preventing their absorption. This can help to reduce the risk of heart disease, stroke, and other chronic health conditions.

Fiber also plays an important role in gut health, as it helps to promote the growth of healthy gut bacteria. These bacteria help to break down fiber into short-chain fatty acids, which provide energy for the cells lining the colon and may have anti-inflammatory effects.

Despite the many benefits of fiber, many people do not consume enough of it. The recommended daily intake of fiber for adults is 25-30 grams, but most Americans consume only about half of that amount. This is largely due to a diet that is high in processed foods and low in fruits, vegetables, and whole grains.

To increase your intake of fiber, try to include a variety of high-fiber foods in your diet, such as berries, leafy greens, beans, and whole grains. Be sure to also drink plenty of water, as fiber needs water to do its job properly. If you are new to consuming high-fiber foods, it is important to increase your intake gradually to avoid digestive discomfort.

In conclusion, fiber plays a critical role in blood sugar regulation and overall health. By slowing down the absorption of glucose into the bloodstream, fiber can help to maintain stable blood sugar levels over time. In addition, fiber has a number of other health benefits, including reducing the risk of heart disease and promoting gut health. To reap the benefits of fiber, it is important to consume a diet that is high in fiber-rich foods, such as fruits, vegetables, and whole grains.

Chapter 8

The Benefits of Probiotics and Gut Health for Blood Sugar Balance

The human body is home to trillions of microorganisms, including bacteria, fungi, and viruses, which make up what is known as the microbiome. The gut microbiome, in particular, plays a critical role in our health, including blood sugar regulation. One key component of the gut microbiome that has been shown to have a significant impact on blood sugar balance is probiotics.

Probiotics are live microorganisms that, when consumed in adequate amounts, confer health benefits to the host. They are found in fermented foods such as yogurt, kefir, and sauerkraut, as well as in probiotic supplements. Probiotics work by promoting the growth of beneficial bacteria in the gut, which can help to improve digestion, boost the immune system, and regulate blood sugar levels.

One of the ways in which probiotics can help to regulate blood sugar levels is by improving insulin sensitivity. Insulin is the hormone that helps to regulate blood sugar levels by allowing glucose to enter cells where it can be used for energy. When cells become resistant to insulin, the body produces more insulin to compensate, leading to higher blood sugar levels over time. Studies have shown that consuming probiotics can improve insulin sensitivity and reduce insulin resistance, which can help to regulate blood sugar levels and reduce the risk of developing type 2 diabetes.

Probiotics can also have an impact on appetite and weight management, which are closely linked to blood sugar regulation. Some studies have shown that consuming probiotics can help to reduce feelings of hunger and increase feelings of fullness, which can help to control food intake and reduce the risk of overeating. In addition, probiotics have been shown to reduce inflammation in the gut, which is associated with obesity and metabolic disorders.

Another way in which probiotics can impact blood sugar regulation is by promoting the production of short-chain fatty acids (SCFAs) in the gut. SCFAs are produced by gut bacteria when they ferment dietary fiber, and they have been shown to improve insulin sensitivity and regulate blood sugar levels. They also play a role in reducing inflammation in the gut and promoting the growth of healthy gut bacteria.

To reap the benefits of probiotics for blood sugar balance, it is important to consume a variety of probiotic-rich foods and supplements. In addition to fermented foods, probiotics can be found in probiotic supplements, which can be taken daily to support gut health. It is also important to consume a diet that is high in fiber, as this provides the food that probiotics need to thrive.

In addition to consuming probiotics, there are other steps that can be taken to support gut health and blood sugar regulation. These include consuming a diet that is rich in fruits, vegetables, and whole grains, as well as reducing intake of processed and high-sugar foods. Regular exercise and stress management techniques, such as meditation and yoga, can also have a positive impact on gut health and blood sugar regulation.

In conclusion, the gut microbiome plays a critical role in blood sugar regulation, and probiotics are an important tool for supporting gut health and blood sugar balance. By improving insulin sensitivity, reducing inflammation, and promoting the growth of healthy gut bacteria, probiotics can help to reduce the risk of developing type 2 diabetes and improve overall health. To reap the benefits of probiotics, it is important to consume a variety of probiotic-rich foods and supplements, as well as to support gut health through a healthy diet, regular exercise, and stress management techniques.

Chapter 9

The Dangers of Processed Foods and Sugar in the Diet

Processed foods and added sugars have become a major part of the modern diet, leading to a significant increase in chronic diseases such as diabetes, obesity, and heart disease. In this chapter, we will discuss the dangers of processed foods and added sugars, and how they can impact blood sugar balance and overall health.

The Rise of Processed Foods and Added Sugars
In the last few decades, the consumption of processed foods and added sugars has increased dramatically. This is due in part to the convenience and affordability of these foods, as well as the aggressive marketing tactics used by the food industry to promote them. Processed foods are typically high in calories, unhealthy fats, salt, and

added sugars, while being low in nutrients such as fiber, vitamins, and minerals.

Impact on Blood Sugar Balance
Processed foods and added sugars can cause a rapid rise in blood sugar levels, leading to a spike in insulin levels, followed by a subsequent drop in blood sugar levels. This rollercoaster effect can lead to a range of health issues, including diabetes, insulin resistance, and metabolic syndrome. Additionally, consuming these foods on a regular basis can cause chronic inflammation, which can contribute to the development of numerous chronic diseases.

The Dangers of Added Sugars
Added sugars are one of the biggest culprits in the rise of chronic diseases. These sugars are added to a wide range of foods, from breakfast cereals and baked goods to soft drinks and condiments. They provide empty calories, with no nutritional value,

and are often added to foods that are already high in calories and unhealthy fats. Consuming too much added sugar can lead to weight gain, type 2 diabetes, and heart disease.

The Dangers of Processed Foods
Processed foods are also a major contributor to chronic disease. These foods are typically high in unhealthy fats, sodium, and calories, and low in fiber, vitamins, and minerals. They often contain artificial additives and preservatives that can have negative effects on health. Additionally, many processed foods are designed to be addictive, making it difficult for individuals to make healthy food choices.

How to Reduce the Consumption of Processed Foods and Added Sugars

Reducing the consumption of processed foods and added sugars is key to achieving optimal health and blood sugar balance. One way to achieve this is by choosing whole, nutrient-dense foods such as fruits, vegetables, whole grains, and lean proteins. These foods provide essential nutrients that support overall health and are less likely to cause a rapid rise in blood sugar levels.

Additionally, individuals can become more aware of the ingredients in their food by reading food labels and avoiding products that contain added sugars or unhealthy fats. They can also choose to cook meals at home using fresh ingredients, which allows for more control over the quality and nutrient content of the food.

Conclusion
Processed foods and added sugars are a major contributor to the rise of chronic diseases such as diabetes, obesity, and heart disease. They can cause

a rapid rise and fall in blood sugar levels, leading to
a range of health issues. By reducing the
consumption of these foods and choosing whole,
nutrient-dense foods, individuals can support
blood sugar balance and overall health.

Chapter 10

The Benefits of Whole Foods and Balanced Nutrition for Optimal Health

Whole foods are foods that are minimally processed and free of artificial ingredients, while balanced nutrition means consuming a variety of nutrients in the right proportions. Both whole foods and balanced nutrition are essential for optimal health, as they provide the body with the necessary nutrients it needs to function properly. In this chapter, we will explore the benefits of whole foods and balanced nutrition, and how they can help maintain blood sugar balance, prevent chronic diseases, and promote overall health.

The Importance of Whole Foods:
Whole foods are foods that are in their natural state, meaning they have not been altered or processed.

These foods are typically high in nutrients such as vitamins, minerals, and fiber, which are essential for optimal health. By consuming whole foods, we can provide our bodies with the necessary nutrients it needs to function properly, while also avoiding the harmful additives and chemicals found in processed foods.

Whole foods are also beneficial for blood sugar balance. These foods are typically low on the glycemic index, which means they do not cause a rapid spike in blood sugar levels. This is important because when blood sugar levels spike, the body produces insulin to regulate it, which can lead to insulin resistance over time. By consuming whole foods, we can help prevent insulin resistance and maintain healthy blood sugar levels.

The Importance of Balanced Nutrition:
Balanced nutrition means consuming a variety of nutrients in the right proportions. This includes

consuming a balance of macronutrients (carbohydrates, proteins, and fats) as well as micronutrients (vitamins and minerals). When we consume a balanced diet, we can provide our bodies with the necessary nutrients it needs to function properly, while also avoiding the negative health consequences associated with nutrient deficiencies.

Balanced nutrition is also important for blood sugar balance. Consuming too many carbohydrates without enough protein and healthy fats can lead to blood sugar spikes and crashes. On the other hand, consuming too much protein without enough carbohydrates can lead to the production of ketones, which can be harmful to the body in large amounts. By consuming a balanced diet, we can help maintain healthy blood sugar levels and prevent chronic diseases such as diabetes.

The Benefits of Whole Foods and Balanced Nutrition for Optimal Health:

Improved Energy Levels: Consuming whole foods and balanced nutrition can help provide the body with the necessary nutrients it needs to function properly, which can lead to increased energy levels.

Improved Digestion: Whole foods are typically high in fiber, which can help improve digestion and prevent constipation. Balanced nutrition can also help promote digestive health by providing the body with the necessary nutrients it needs to support digestive function.

Weight Management: Consuming whole foods and balanced nutrition can help promote weight management by providing the body with the necessary nutrients it needs to function properly, while also preventing overconsumption of unhealthy foods.

Disease Prevention: Consuming whole foods and balanced nutrition can help prevent chronic diseases such as heart disease, diabetes, and cancer by providing the body with the necessary nutrients it needs to function properly.

Improved Mental Health: Consuming whole foods and balanced nutrition can help improve mental health by providing the body with the necessary nutrients it needs to support brain function, while also preventing the negative health consequences associated with nutrient deficiencies.

Conclusion:
Whole foods and balanced nutrition are essential for optimal health. By consuming a diet rich in whole foods and balanced nutrition, we can provide our bodies with the necessary nutrients it needs to function properly, while also preventing chronic diseases and promoting overall health. To maintain blood sugar balance and achieve optimal health, it is

important to prioritize whole foods and balanced
nutrition in our diets.

Chapter 11

Fasting and Intermittent Fasting: A Tool for Achieving Blood Sugar Balance

Fasting and intermittent fasting have been gaining popularity in recent years for their potential health benefits. Fasting is the practice of abstaining from food or drink for a period of time, while intermittent fasting involves alternating periods of eating and fasting. Both have been shown to have a positive impact on blood sugar regulation, making them powerful tools in achieving optimal health.

Understanding Fasting and Intermittent Fasting

Fasting has been practiced for thousands of years for religious, spiritual, and health reasons. In recent years, it has gained popularity as a tool for weight loss and improving metabolic health. Intermittent fasting is a variation of fasting that involves alternating periods of eating and fasting. The most popular methods of intermittent fasting include the 16/8 method, where you fast for 16 hours and eat during an 8-hour window, and the 5:2 method, where you eat normally for 5 days and restrict calorie intake to 500-600 for 2 non-consecutive days.

Benefits of Fasting and Intermittent Fasting for Blood Sugar Balance
Fasting and intermittent fasting have been shown to have numerous benefits for blood sugar balance, including:

Improved Insulin Sensitivity: Fasting and intermittent fasting have been shown to improve insulin sensitivity, allowing the body to use insulin more effectively and maintain healthy blood sugar levels.

Reduced Insulin Resistance: Insulin resistance is a condition where the body becomes less responsive to insulin, leading to high blood sugar levels. Fasting and intermittent fasting have been shown to reduce insulin resistance and improve blood sugar control.

Increased Autophagy: Autophagy is the process by which the body breaks down and recycles old or damaged cells. Fasting and intermittent fasting have been shown to increase autophagy, which may help improve insulin sensitivity and blood sugar control.

Weight Loss: Fasting and intermittent fasting have been shown to promote weight loss, which can help improve blood sugar control and reduce the risk of type 2 diabetes.

Reduced Inflammation: Chronic inflammation is linked to insulin resistance and poor blood sugar control. Fasting and intermittent fasting have been shown to reduce inflammation, improving blood sugar balance.

Improved Gut Health: Fasting and intermittent fasting have been shown to improve gut health by promoting the growth of beneficial gut bacteria and reducing inflammation in the gut.

Reduced Oxidative Stress: Oxidative stress is a condition where there is an imbalance between free radicals and antioxidants in the body, leading to cell damage. Fasting and intermittent fasting have been shown to reduce oxidative stress, improving overall health and blood sugar control.

How to Incorporate Fasting and Intermittent Fasting into Your Lifestyle

If you are interested in trying fasting or intermittent fasting, it is important to do so safely and with guidance from a healthcare professional. Here are some tips to help you get started:

Start Slowly: If you are new to fasting or intermittent fasting, start with shorter fasts or try the 16/8 method before moving on to more advanced methods.

Stay Hydrated: During a fast or period of restricted calorie intake, it is important to stay hydrated by drinking plenty of water and electrolyte-rich fluids.

Listen to Your Body: If you experience dizziness, weakness, or other symptoms during a fast, it is important to listen to your body and break the fast if necessary.

Break Your Fast with Healthy Foods: When breaking a fast, it is important to choose nutrient-dense, whole foods to support blood sugar balance and overall health.

Seek Professional Guidance: If you have a medical condition or are taking medication, it is important

Chapter 12

The Importance of Quality Sleep for Blood Sugar Balance and Overall Health

Sleep is often overlooked when it comes to overall health and wellness. However, the impact of sleep on our bodies and minds cannot be overstated. Sleep is essential for regulating various bodily functions, including blood sugar levels. In this chapter, we will explore the importance of quality sleep for blood sugar balance and overall health.

The Link Between Sleep and Blood Sugar
Studies have shown that sleep deprivation and poor sleep quality can lead to insulin resistance, a condition where the body's cells become less responsive to insulin. Insulin resistance makes it harder for the body to regulate blood sugar levels, leading to higher levels of glucose in the bloodstream. This, in turn, can lead to a range of

health problems, including type 2 diabetes, obesity, and cardiovascular disease.

In addition, sleep deprivation can also lead to an increase in the stress hormone cortisol, which can raise blood sugar levels. Cortisol is typically highest in the morning and gradually decreases throughout the day. However, when we don't get enough sleep, cortisol levels can remain elevated throughout the day, leading to increased blood sugar levels.

The Role of Melatonin
Melatonin is a hormone produced by the body that helps regulate sleep-wake cycles. It also has a role in regulating blood sugar levels. Studies have shown that melatonin can improve insulin sensitivity and glucose tolerance, leading to better blood sugar regulation. Melatonin has also been shown to have anti-inflammatory properties, which can help reduce the risk of developing chronic diseases such as diabetes.

The Importance of Circadian Rhythms
Our bodies have an internal clock, known as the circadian rhythm, which regulates various bodily functions, including sleep and blood sugar levels. Disrupting the circadian rhythm, such as by staying up late or working night shifts, can lead to an imbalance in blood sugar levels.

Research has shown that individuals who work night shifts are at an increased risk of developing metabolic disorders, including obesity and type 2 diabetes. This is because working at night disrupts the body's natural circadian rhythm, leading to an imbalance in hormones that regulate blood sugar levels.

Tips for Improving Sleep Quality
Improving sleep quality can have a significant impact on blood sugar regulation and overall health. Here are some tips for getting better sleep:

Stick to a regular sleep schedule: Try to go to bed and wake up at the same time every day, even on weekends.

Create a relaxing sleep environment: Make sure your bedroom is cool, dark, and quiet. Use blackout curtains or a sleep mask to block out any light.

Avoid stimulating activities before bed: Avoid using electronic devices, watching TV, or engaging in stimulating activities before bed.

Exercise regularly: Regular exercise can improve sleep quality and regulate blood sugar levels.

Limit caffeine and alcohol: Caffeine and alcohol can disrupt sleep, so it's best to limit their consumption, especially before bed.

Practice relaxation techniques: Techniques such as deep breathing, meditation, and yoga can help promote relaxation and improve sleep quality.

Conclusion
Quality sleep is essential for regulating various bodily functions, including blood sugar levels. Disrupting the circadian rhythm through poor sleep habits can lead to an imbalance in hormones that regulate blood sugar levels, leading to an increased risk of developing chronic diseases such as diabetes. By prioritizing sleep and making simple changes to improve sleep quality, individuals can improve blood sugar regulation and overall health.

Chapter 13

The Importance of Hydration for Blood Sugar Balance and Overall Health

Water is the foundation of all life, and our bodies are made up of around 60% water. It is essential for the proper functioning of all our bodily systems, including the regulation of blood sugar levels. In fact, dehydration can lead to imbalances in blood sugar levels and contribute to a host of health problems.

Dehydration and Blood Sugar Levels
When we become dehydrated, the concentration of sugar in our blood increases, leading to higher blood sugar levels. This is because the kidneys are responsible for regulating the balance of fluids and electrolytes in our bodies, and when we become dehydrated, they start to retain water to maintain

the balance of fluids in the body. This can cause the blood sugar levels to become imbalanced and can contribute to the development of diabetes.

Dehydration can also impair insulin sensitivity, which means that our cells are less able to respond to insulin and take up glucose from the bloodstream. This can lead to higher blood sugar levels and increase the risk of developing type 2 diabetes.

The Importance of Hydration
Drinking enough water throughout the day is essential for maintaining proper blood sugar levels and overall health. The recommended daily intake of water is around 2-3 liters for adults, but this can vary depending on factors such as age, sex, activity level, and climate.

In addition to water, certain foods and drinks can also help with hydration. Fruits and vegetables, for example, are high in water content and can help keep us hydrated. Herbal teas, coconut water, and low-sugar sports drinks can also be good options for staying hydrated.

Benefits of Proper Hydration
In addition to regulating blood sugar levels, staying properly hydrated has a host of other health benefits. It helps to:

Maintain healthy skin
Aid in digestion
Regulate body temperature
Keep joints lubricated
Flush toxins from the body
Tips for Staying Hydrated

Here are some tips to help you stay hydrated throughout the day:
Drink water regularly throughout the day: Carry a reusable water bottle with you and sip on water regularly.

Eat hydrating foods: Fruits and vegetables, such as watermelon, cucumbers, and celery, are high in water content and can help keep you hydrated.

Limit sugary and caffeinated drinks: Drinks like soda, energy drinks, and coffee can actually dehydrate you, so it's best to limit your intake of these beverages.

Drink water before, during, and after exercise: It's important to stay hydrated during physical activity, so make sure to drink water before, during, and after your workout.

Monitor your urine color: Urine color is a good indicator of hydration levels. If your urine is dark yellow or amber, it's a sign that you need to drink more water.

In conclusion, proper hydration is essential for maintaining healthy blood sugar levels and overall health. Drinking enough water and staying hydrated throughout the day can help regulate blood sugar levels, improve insulin sensitivity, and reduce the risk of developing diabetes. It's important to make staying hydrated a priority in your daily routine to optimize your health and well-being.

Chapter 14

The Benefits of Herbs and Spices for Blood Sugar Balance

Herbs and spices have been used for centuries to enhance the flavor of food, but they also have medicinal properties that can improve our health. In recent years, there has been increasing interest in the use of herbs and spices for blood sugar balance, and for good reason. Studies have shown that certain herbs and spices have the ability to lower blood sugar levels, reduce insulin resistance, and improve glucose tolerance.

In this chapter, we will explore some of the most promising herbs and spices for blood sugar balance and how they work.

Cinnamon

Cinnamon is a popular spice that has been shown to improve insulin sensitivity and lower fasting blood sugar levels. Cinnamon contains bioactive compounds that have been found to mimic insulin and improve glucose uptake in the cells. Studies have also shown that cinnamon can reduce inflammation in the body, which can contribute to insulin resistance.

Ginger

Ginger is another spice that has been shown to have anti-inflammatory properties and can help improve insulin sensitivity. A study published in the journal Complementary Therapies in Medicine found that ginger supplementation reduced fasting blood sugar levels and improved insulin sensitivity in people with type 2 diabetes.

Turmeric

Turmeric is a bright yellow spice that is widely used
in Indian cuisine. It contains a compound called
curcumin, which has been found to have
anti-inflammatory and antioxidant properties.
Studies have shown that curcumin can improve
insulin sensitivity and glucose uptake in the cells. A
study published in the Journal of Diabetes Science
and Technology found that curcumin
supplementation improved blood sugar control and
reduced inflammation in people with type 2
diabetes.

Fenugreek

Fenugreek is an herb that is commonly used in
Indian and Middle Eastern cuisine. It has been
shown to improve insulin sensitivity and lower
fasting blood sugar levels. A study published in the
Journal of Diabetes and its Complications found
that fenugreek supplementation improved glucose

tolerance and reduced insulin resistance in people with type 2 diabetes.

Garlic

Garlic is a common herb that is used in many different cuisines. It has been found to have numerous health benefits, including blood sugar regulation. Studies have shown that garlic supplementation can improve insulin sensitivity and reduce fasting blood sugar levels. A study published in the Journal of Medicinal Food found that garlic extract supplementation improved glucose control and reduced oxidative stress in people with type 2 diabetes.

Rosemary

Rosemary is a fragrant herb that is commonly used in Mediterranean cuisine. It contains carnosic acid, a compound that has been found to have antioxidant and anti-inflammatory properties.

Studies have shown that rosemary extract can improve glucose tolerance and lower fasting blood sugar levels in people with type 2 diabetes.

Conclusion

Herbs and spices are a great way to add flavor to your food while also reaping the benefits of their medicinal properties. Incorporating these herbs and spices into your diet can help improve blood sugar regulation and reduce the risk of developing type 2 diabetes. While herbs and spices can be a helpful addition to your blood sugar management plan, it's important to remember that they are not a substitute for a healthy diet and regular exercise. As always, it's important to talk to your healthcare provider before making any changes to your diet or lifestyle.

Chapter 15

Blood Sugar Balance and Hormonal Health: The Connection Between Insulin and Other Hormones

Hormones play a crucial role in regulating many bodily functions, including blood sugar control. Insulin, one of the most important hormones involved in blood sugar regulation, works in concert with other hormones to maintain proper blood sugar levels. Hormonal imbalances can lead to blood sugar dysregulation and a host of other health issues. In this chapter, we will explore the relationship between insulin and other hormones, and how they work together to promote blood sugar balance and overall health.

Insulin and Blood Sugar Control
Insulin is a hormone produced by the pancreas that helps regulate blood sugar levels. After we eat a meal, our body breaks down carbohydrates into glucose, which enters the bloodstream. The pancreas then releases insulin, which helps move glucose from the blood into the cells, where it can be used for energy or stored for later use.

When blood sugar levels are consistently high, the body can become less sensitive to insulin, which can lead to insulin resistance. Insulin resistance is a condition in which the body produces insulin but is unable to use it effectively, resulting in high blood sugar levels. This can eventually lead to prediabetes or type 2 diabetes.

Other Hormones and Blood Sugar Regulation
While insulin is the primary hormone involved in blood sugar regulation, it works in conjunction with other hormones to maintain balance. One of

these hormones is glucagon, which is produced by the pancreas and raises blood sugar levels when they are too low. Glucagon signals the liver to release stored glucose into the bloodstream, providing the body with an additional source of energy.

Another hormone involved in blood sugar regulation is cortisol, which is produced by the adrenal glands in response to stress. Cortisol raises blood sugar levels by increasing the production of glucose in the liver. However, chronically elevated cortisol levels due to chronic stress can lead to insulin resistance and blood sugar dysregulation.

Thyroid hormones, which are produced by the thyroid gland, also play a role in blood sugar regulation. They affect the body's metabolic rate and can influence how quickly glucose is taken up by cells.

Estrogen and progesterone, two female sex hormones, also affect blood sugar regulation. Estrogen can increase insulin sensitivity and promote glucose uptake, while progesterone can decrease insulin sensitivity.

Imbalances in any of these hormones can lead to blood sugar dysregulation and increased risk of chronic disease.

The Connection Between Insulin Resistance and Other Hormonal Imbalances
Insulin resistance is often associated with other hormonal imbalances. For example, women with polycystic ovary syndrome (PCOS) often have insulin resistance as well as imbalances in estrogen and progesterone. In men, insulin resistance can lead to decreased testosterone production, which can further exacerbate blood sugar dysregulation.

Chronic stress and elevated cortisol levels can also contribute to insulin resistance, as well as imbalances in other hormones. For example, chronically elevated cortisol levels can suppress thyroid function, leading to decreased thyroid hormone production and slower metabolic rate.

Addressing Hormonal Imbalances for Blood Sugar Balance
Maintaining healthy hormonal balance is essential for optimal blood sugar control and overall health. Eating a balanced diet that includes healthy fats, protein, and fiber can help regulate blood sugar and support hormonal health.

Reducing stress through mindfulness practices such as meditation, yoga, or deep breathing can also help balance hormones and promote blood sugar regulation. Adequate sleep, regular exercise, and staying hydrated are also important for maintaining hormonal balance and optimal blood sugar control.

In some cases, targeted supplementation may be necessary to address hormonal imbalances. For example, women with PCOS may benefit from supplements such as inositol, which can improve insulin sensitivity and promote hormonal balance.

While insulin plays a crucial role in blood sugar balance, it is not the only hormone involved. Hormones such as cortisol, estrogen, progesterone, testosterone, and thyroid hormones also play important roles in blood sugar regulation.

Cortisol, often referred to as the "stress hormone," is released in response to stress and can cause blood sugar levels to rise. When cortisol levels remain elevated for extended periods, it can lead to insulin resistance and diabetes. Estrogen and progesterone can also impact insulin sensitivity, with estrogen increasing sensitivity and progesterone decreasing it.

Testosterone can also play a role in insulin sensitivity, with low testosterone levels linked to insulin resistance and diabetes. Thyroid hormones can also impact blood sugar regulation, with an underactive thyroid (hypothyroidism) associated with insulin resistance and an increased risk of diabetes.

In addition to insulin, these hormones work together to maintain blood sugar balance in the body. Any disruption in their levels or function can lead to imbalances in blood sugar levels and increase the risk of developing diabetes and other chronic diseases.

Fortunately, there are several lifestyle changes that can help support hormonal balance and promote healthy blood sugar levels. This includes a balanced diet, regular exercise, stress management techniques, and good sleep hygiene.

Certain dietary and lifestyle factors can also help support hormonal balance. Eating a diet rich in fiber, whole foods, and healthy fats can help regulate hormones and promote blood sugar balance. Regular exercise and stress management techniques such as meditation and yoga can also help regulate cortisol levels and promote hormonal balance.

Additionally, getting adequate sleep and maintaining good sleep hygiene can help regulate hormone levels, including insulin. Aim for at least 7-8 hours of quality sleep each night, and establish a regular sleep schedule to support hormonal balance.

In summary, insulin is not the only hormone involved in blood sugar regulation. Hormones such as cortisol, estrogen, progesterone, testosterone, and thyroid hormones also play important roles in maintaining healthy blood sugar levels. Lifestyle factors such as diet, exercise, stress management, and sleep hygiene can all help support hormonal balance and promote optimal blood sugar regulation.

Chapter 16

Blood Sugar Imbalance and Chronic Disease: The Link Between High Blood Sugar and Conditions like Diabetes, Cardiovascular Disease, and Cancer

Blood sugar imbalance is a condition that can lead to a number of chronic diseases, including diabetes, cardiovascular disease, and cancer. When the body is unable to properly regulate blood sugar levels, it can have a serious impact on overall health.

One of the most significant risks of blood sugar imbalance is the development of type 2 diabetes. In this condition, the body becomes resistant to the effects of insulin, which is the hormone responsible for regulating blood sugar levels. As a result, blood sugar levels can become dangerously high, leading to a range of symptoms and complications.

Diabetes is a major cause of cardiovascular disease, which is the leading cause of death worldwide. High blood sugar can damage blood vessels and increase the risk of heart attack, stroke, and other cardiovascular problems. It can also lead to kidney disease, nerve damage, and blindness.

Cancer is another disease that has been linked to blood sugar imbalance. Researchers have found that high blood sugar levels can fuel the growth of cancer cells, increasing the risk of developing certain types of cancer.

Fortunately, there are steps that can be taken to help prevent blood sugar imbalance and reduce the risk of chronic disease. One of the most important strategies is maintaining a healthy diet. This means avoiding processed and sugary foods, and instead focusing on whole, nutrient-dense foods that can help regulate blood sugar levels.

Regular exercise is also key to maintaining healthy blood sugar levels. Exercise can help increase insulin sensitivity, allowing the body to use glucose more effectively. It can also help burn excess glucose in the bloodstream, reducing the risk of complications associated with high blood sugar levels.

In addition to diet and exercise, stress management is another important factor in maintaining healthy blood sugar levels. Chronic stress can have a negative impact on insulin sensitivity and increase the risk of blood sugar imbalance. Strategies like meditation, yoga, and deep breathing exercises can be effective in reducing stress and promoting overall health.

Taking steps to improve gut health and microbiome diversity can also be helpful in regulating blood sugar levels. Consuming probiotic-rich foods like yogurt and kefir, as well as prebiotic-rich foods like onions, garlic, and asparagus, can promote healthy gut bacteria and reduce the risk of blood sugar imbalance.

Finally, it's important to be proactive about monitoring blood sugar levels and addressing any imbalances that arise. Regular check-ups with a healthcare provider, as well as monitoring blood sugar levels at home using a glucometer, can help identify any issues and allow for prompt treatment.

In summary, blood sugar imbalance can have a significant impact on overall health, and can increase the risk of chronic disease like diabetes, cardiovascular disease, and cancer. However, by maintaining a healthy diet, engaging in regular exercise, managing stress, promoting gut health, and monitoring blood sugar levels, it is possible to reduce the risk of complications and maintain optimal health.

Chapter 17

The Benefits of Blood Sugar Monitoring: Tools and Techniques for Tracking Blood Sugar Levels

Blood sugar monitoring is an essential tool for achieving and maintaining optimal health. By tracking your blood sugar levels, you can gain a better understanding of how different foods, lifestyle habits, and medications affect your body's ability to regulate blood sugar. In this chapter, we will explore the benefits of blood sugar monitoring, different techniques and tools for tracking blood sugar levels, and how to interpret the results.

Why Monitor Blood Sugar?
Monitoring blood sugar levels is important for several reasons. First and foremost, it allows you to identify patterns in your blood sugar levels and make changes to your diet and lifestyle to keep your

blood sugar within a healthy range. This is particularly important for people with diabetes, who need to monitor their blood sugar levels closely to prevent complications.

Monitoring blood sugar levels can also help identify early warning signs of diabetes or other health problems, such as high blood pressure, high cholesterol, or cardiovascular disease. By catching these conditions early, you can take steps to prevent or manage them before they become more serious.

Tools for Monitoring Blood Sugar
There are several tools available for monitoring blood sugar levels, including blood glucose meters, continuous glucose monitors, and urine glucose tests.

Blood glucose meters are handheld devices that measure blood sugar levels from a small drop of blood taken from your fingertip. These meters are easy to use and provide quick results, but they require regular finger pricks and can be less accurate than other methods.

Continuous glucose monitors (CGMs) are wearable devices that measure blood sugar levels continuously throughout the day. These devices use a small sensor inserted under the skin to measure glucose levels in the interstitial fluid, which is the fluid that surrounds cells in the body. CGMs provide real-time data on blood sugar levels and can be particularly helpful for people with diabetes who need to closely monitor their blood sugar levels.

Urine glucose tests are another option for monitoring blood sugar levels. These tests use special strips that change color in response to glucose in the urine. While urine glucose tests can provide a general idea of blood sugar levels, they are less accurate than other methods and are not recommended for people with diabetes.

Interpreting Blood Sugar Results

When monitoring blood sugar levels, it's important to know what the results mean. In general, a healthy blood sugar range is between 70 and 140 mg/dL, although this can vary depending on factors such as age, weight, and overall health.

If your blood sugar levels are consistently outside of this range, it may be a sign of an underlying health problem, such as diabetes or prediabetes. In this case, it's important to speak with your healthcare provider about developing a plan to manage your blood sugar levels.

In addition to monitoring your blood sugar levels, it's important to pay attention to other factors that can affect blood sugar, such as diet, exercise, stress, and medication. By making lifestyle changes and

working with your healthcare provider, you can
maintain healthy blood sugar levels and reduce your
risk of chronic diseases.

Conclusion

Monitoring blood sugar levels is an essential tool for
achieving and maintaining optimal health. By
tracking your blood sugar levels, you can identify
patterns and make changes to your diet and lifestyle
to keep your blood sugar within a healthy range.
There are several tools available for monitoring
blood sugar levels, including blood glucose meters,
continuous glucose monitors, and urine glucose
tests. It's important to interpret blood sugar results
in the context of other factors that can affect blood
sugar levels, such as diet, exercise, stress, and
medication. With regular monitoring and proper
management, you can maintain healthy blood sugar
levels and reduce your risk of chronic diseases.

Chapter 18

Practical Tips for Achieving and Maintaining Blood Sugar Balance in Daily Life

Maintaining blood sugar balance is essential for good health, and it is a lifelong process that requires consistent effort and attention. In this chapter, we will explore some practical tips for achieving and maintaining blood sugar balance in daily life.

Choose Whole Foods

One of the best ways to achieve blood sugar balance is to eat whole, nutrient-dense foods. These include vegetables, fruits, whole grains, lean proteins, and healthy fats. Processed foods, on the other hand, are often high in sugar and refined carbohydrates, which can cause blood sugar spikes and crashes. When you eat whole foods, you're giving your body the nutrients it needs to function properly and maintain healthy blood sugar levels.

Pay Attention to Portion Sizes

Another key to blood sugar balance is eating appropriate portion sizes. Even healthy foods can cause blood sugar spikes if you eat too much of them. The American Diabetes Association recommends using a plate method for meal planning: fill half your plate with non-starchy vegetables, one quarter with lean protein, and one quarter with a starchy carbohydrate.

Keep Carbohydrate Intake in Check

Carbohydrates are one of the primary sources of glucose in the body, so it's important to be mindful of how many carbohydrates you eat. This doesn't mean you need to cut carbs out of your diet entirely, but it does mean paying attention to the types and amounts of carbs you consume. Choose complex carbs, like whole grains, fruits, and

vegetables, and limit simple carbs, like candy and
sugary drinks.

Incorporate Protein and Healthy Fats into Your
Meals
Protein and healthy fats can help slow down the
absorption of glucose into the bloodstream, which
can prevent blood sugar spikes. Incorporate sources
of protein and healthy fats into your meals, like
nuts, seeds, avocado, fish, and chicken. This can
help you feel fuller longer and stabilize your blood
sugar levels.

Stay Hydrated
Drinking plenty of water is important for
maintaining healthy blood sugar levels. When
you're dehydrated, your blood becomes thicker and
more concentrated, which can lead to higher blood
sugar levels. Aim for at least eight glasses of water a
day, and try to limit your intake of sugary drinks,
which can cause blood sugar spikes.

Get Moving

Regular exercise can help improve insulin
sensitivity, which can improve blood sugar control.
Aim for at least 30 minutes of moderate-intensity
exercise most days of the week, like brisk walking,
cycling, or swimming. If you're new to exercise,
start slowly and work your way up to longer and
more intense workouts.

Practice Stress-Reducing Techniques

Stress can cause blood sugar spikes, so it's important
to find ways to manage stress in your life. This
could include techniques like meditation, deep
breathing, yoga, or spending time in nature.
Experiment with different techniques and find
what works best for you.

Monitor Your Blood Sugar Levels

Regular blood sugar monitoring can help you stay
on top of your blood sugar levels and make

adjustments as needed. Talk to your healthcare provider about how often you should be checking your blood sugar and what your target ranges should be.

Work with a Healthcare Provider
If you're struggling to achieve and maintain blood sugar balance, consider working with a healthcare provider who specializes in blood sugar management. They can help you develop a personalized plan that takes into account your unique needs and goals.

In conclusion, achieving and maintaining blood sugar balance is an important part of overall health and wellness. By incorporating these practical tips into your daily life, you can help keep your blood sugar levels stable and reduce your risk of chronic disease. Remember that it's a lifelong journey, so be patient and persistent in your efforts to achieve and maintain optimal blood sugar balance.

Conclusion

The Sweet Spot of Optimal Health Through Blood Sugar Balance

Congratulations! You have made it to the end of this book on blood sugar balance and its impact on health. Through the course of this book, we have explored a variety of topics related to blood sugar regulation, including the glycemic index, insulin resistance, exercise, stress, fiber, probiotics, processed foods, hydration, herbs and spices, hormonal health, chronic disease, blood sugar monitoring, and practical tips for achieving and maintaining blood sugar balance in daily life.

All of these topics are crucial components in the journey toward optimal health, and the importance of blood sugar balance cannot be overstated. As we have seen, maintaining healthy blood sugar levels can have a significant impact on overall health and well-being, from improving energy and mood to reducing the risk of chronic diseases such as diabetes, cardiovascular disease, and cancer.

By understanding the science behind blood sugar regulation, we can make informed choices about the foods we eat, the lifestyle habits we adopt, and the supplements we take to support our health. We can also develop a deeper appreciation for the interconnectedness of the body's systems and the ways in which they work together to maintain balance and harmony.

As with any journey, achieving and maintaining optimal health requires commitment, effort, and discipline. It may take time to establish new habits and overcome old ones, but the rewards of a balanced blood sugar and optimal health are well worth the effort.

Here are some key takeaways to remember:

Understand the glycemic index and choose foods that have a lower glycemic index to help regulate blood sugar levels.

Exercise regularly to help maintain healthy blood sugar levels, reduce insulin resistance, and improve overall health.

Manage stress through relaxation techniques, mindfulness practices, and regular physical activity to help reduce cortisol levels and support healthy blood sugar levels.

Consume adequate fiber and hydrate regularly to support gut health, reduce inflammation, and maintain healthy blood sugar levels.

Incorporate probiotics into your diet to support gut health and improve blood sugar regulation.

Avoid processed foods and added sugars, which can contribute to insulin resistance and chronic diseases.

Monitor your blood sugar levels regularly to identify patterns and make adjustments to your diet and lifestyle as needed.

Practice mindful eating to help regulate blood sugar levels and support healthy digestion.

By incorporating these principles into our daily lives, we can achieve the sweet spot of optimal health through blood sugar balance. We can experience greater vitality, resilience, and joy in all aspects of our lives.

Thank you for taking the time to read this book, and I wish you all the best on your journey toward optimal health and well-being!